BEN CORNICH

30 DAYS WEIGHT LOSS CHALLENGE

Contents

1

INTRODUCTION

You absolutely have the right to feel strong and comfortable in your body. There is nothing wrong with wanting to tone up or lose weight. However, let's be clear: weight loss does not necessarily require strict diets, excessive exercise, or negative self-talk. In fact, you will want to do the exact opposite if you want to lose weight in a healthy and long-lasting way! Forget the self-doubt, long workouts, and tedious calorie counting. And please, do not succumb to fad diets or weight loss products endorsed by social media. Instead, treat your body well. Eat healthy foods, exercise because it makes you feel good both physically and mentally, and show yourself grace and gratitude. In any case, research demonstrates that restrictive diets cannot last for long! So, if you want to lose weight and keep it off, you should take a healthy, slow approach.

How can you begin a healthy and long-lasting weight loss strategy?

Excellent query. Our 30-day weight loss challenge is here! This challenge has a lot of easy-to-follow advice that will make you feel great inside and out. There are no restrictions, tricks, or quick fixes! By teaching you healthy routines that you can incorporate into your daily life, this challenge is merely designed to get you started on your weight loss journey. Because reducing stress, getting enough water, and getting enough sleep are all important factors in weight loss! Therefore, this challenge is not just about losing weight. It involves making a commitment to being healthier.

2

HEIGHT AND WEIGHT

Being overweight or obese makes us more likely to get a lot of diseases. Around 75% of Australian men, 60% of Australian women, and 25% of Australian children are overweight or obese. As a result, obesity-related diseases like diabetes and coronary heart disease are also on the rise.

Weight loss

is now a multi-billion dollar business. It's hard to go a day without reading or hearing about a weight-loss "miracle" or "the answer to."

Making small, healthy changes to your eating and exercise routines is the sensible way to lose weight. If you want to lose weight and keep it off, these changes should be things you can implement into your daily life.

Diet don't work long-term

There are many myths about weight loss. Fad diets and magical weight loss pills endorsed by celebrities and supported by personal success stories abound in popular media. While some of these diets may help you lose weight while you are on them, once you return to your normal routine, the weight begins to come back on. This is due to the fact that maintaining weight loss over time is more challenging than just losing weight.

Not just following a diet for a few weeks to lose weight, but managing your weight is a commitment for the rest of your life.

Keep in mind that you will probably regain any weight you lose if the methods you are using to lose weight are not ones that you will be able to stick with for the rest of your life.

Risk of dieting

Dieting has risks because it causes our bodies to slow down their metabolism in response to semi-starvation.

Fat and muscle are lost when you lose weight too quickly. Unlike fat, muscle burns kilojoules. Because of the decreased proportion of muscle in your body and the slower metabolic rate, your body will burn even fewer calories when you stop dieting and resume your regular routine.

This eating pattern can also have a negative impact on our overall health; even a single cycle of weight loss and gain can increase our risk of coronary heart disease, regardless of our body fat percentage.

5

Because of this, being able to maintain weight loss is more crucial. A weekly weight loss of between 12 and 1 kilogram is considered reasonable and more likely to be sustained.

3

HOW TO START LOSING WEIGHT

There is a lot of information out there, and it is easy to get overwhelmed. If you want to lose weight, a good place to start is with the Australian Guide to Healthy Eating.

If you have been on crash diets for a long time or are having trouble sticking to them, a dietitian can help you lose weight if you are able to avoid unplanned or habitual eating and stick to regular meals and snacks. Dietitians can direct you toward a healthy diet based on the most recent research and customized to your health and lifestyle.

Before beginning any physical activity, consult your doctor if you are overweight, older than 40, or haven't exercised regularly in a long   time.

4

30 DAYS AND 30 HEALTHY HABITS TO LAST A LONG TIME :LOSING WEIGHT NATURALLY

Day 1: Step one: Identify Your Weight Loss Objectives Set goals for losing weight! You need to know your "why" before you start this weight loss journey. Be patient with this. What motivates you to lose weight? Do you want to feel more confident in your body and stronger? Do you want to improve your current symptoms or lower your risk of developing a chronic illness? You, not your friend, neighbor, or that social media influencer you admire, should be the focus of these objectives. This is where you go!

You'll notice that we didn't tell you to set a weight loss goal. Why? Again, because this is a journey. Having a target number can be helpful for some. If that describes you, feel free to include this! For some, it's simple to become fixated on reaching your goal weight and overlook all of your other progress. Remember: The time of day, how hydrated you are, what you eat, and, for women, where you are in your cycle can all affect your weight. Therefore, instead, give it a shot and see how it feels to set your goals around your "why"

Day 2: Perform a comprehensive inventory of your kitchen, refrigerator, and pantry first. Make a list of the foods you have on hand and toss any items that have expired. Also, make sure to read the labels on the ingredients! Consider which products are made with healthy ingredients and which contain sneaky sugars, oils, and additives. After that, take a quick look at everything you have and determine the ratio of unhealthy food to junk food.

We are not advising you to throw away anything unhealthy, but you should try to be careful with the foods you keep. Products won't likely help you achieve your weight loss goals if they are packed with ingredients you can't identify. Make a list of everything that is missing or needs to be restocked, and toss or donate anything that doesn't serve you or your needs!

Day 3: Fill Your Refrigerator Now that your pantry is organized, it's time to stock your kitchen with nutrient-dense foods! However, prior to going to the grocery store, consume a meal or snack! An easy way to lose weight: Don't go shopping hungry! Based on your cravings, according to research, you'll buy foods with more calories and even be more likely to spend more than usual.

Instead, stock your refrigerator with nutritious staples like:

Seasonal produce (considering the Dirty Dozen and Clean) as well as healthy pasta alternatives (such as chickpea and lentil!) are all healthy canned goods.

Day 4: Frozen fruits and vegetables, which are less expensive and just as nutritious, as well as whole grains and complex carbohydrates like quinoa and sweet potatoes Make drinking water a regular part of your morning routine and start your day with a glass! Remember: Changes that last for a long time are the result of taking small, manageable steps. Despite its apparent simplicity, this habit sets the tone for your entire day! Additionally, research suggests that starting your day with a glass of water can help you kick start your metabolism and even cut down on the number of calories you consume each day.

Additionally, since coffee is a diuretic, starting with water can help prevent dehydration if you drink coffee.

You can make a warm herbal tea with it, add lemon, or just drink it plain! Include this healthy trick today, but try to make it a daily no-brainer as well.

Day 5: Make Dinner at Home Can you say that tonight you will make dinner at home? What about during the challenge itself? It may appear daunting, but with a little preparation and knowledge, it is much easier to manage than you might think! What's the deal? utilizing methods like one-pan meals, meal prep, and batch cooking. When you make dinner at home, you have more control over the ingredients. By incorporating nourishing whole-food ingredients into your recipes, you can avoid all those sneaky sugars, oils, and sodium.

And just so you know, many Fit On PRO dinners only require a few ingredients, a short amount of time to cook, or minimal preparation!

Some of our favorites are listed here.

Dinners Prepared in a One-Pot, Baking Sheet, or Pan:

Broccoli Pesto & Cheese Quesadillas Zucchini Parmesan Boats Creamy Tuscan White Bean & Artichoke Skillet One-Pan Herb Crusted Salmon with Sweet Potatoes and Greens One-Pot Vegetarian Lentil Curry Simple Sheet Pan Tofu Fajitas Quick and Easy Options: On the Table in Ten Minutes Lemon Pepper Shrimp and Roasted Broccoli Asian Noodle Salad with Creamy Almond Dressing

Day 6: Walk Five Minutes More Each Day Make a resolution to walk five minutes more each day—that's it! Walk another five minutes if you had planned to walk to the coffee shop. Add a five-minute cool-down walk to the end of your workout if you went for a run. And if all you have time for is a five-minute walk because your schedule is packed, that's also great! This is all about making these five extra minutes count. Again, even though it may not seem like much, it adds up! If you add five extra minutes to your scheduled time each day, that equates to 35 extra minutes per week and 140 extra minutes per month. In addition, it ensures daily activity, even if it is only for five minutes.

Day 7: Make Breakfast a Priority If you are cutting out breakfast in an effort to lose weight, you might want to reevaluate your decision. According to research, skipping breakfast increases the likelihood of weight gain. Moreover, breakfast is the most important meal of the day! Smoothies, eggs, oat bowls, pancakes—what else could be better?

One of the best things you can do for your mind and body is to start your day with a nutritious breakfast. A nutritious breakfast not only provides you with the energy and nutrients you need to start your day, but it also aids in the reduction of cravings and increases satiety, according to research.

Even in the busiest of mornings, these weight loss-friendly suggestions work:

Greek or coconut yogurt, frozen or fresh berries, and a drizzle of nut butter make a protein-packed yogurt bowl.

Add a handful of greens, any leftover pre-cooked vegetables, and some fresh or dried herbs to some scrambled eggs. Serve with a piece of fruit and an avocado!

For a quick and easy breakfast packed with protein, heat up a 2-Minute Blueberry Oatmeal Muffin.

Blend your favorite vegetables, fruits, greens, and super foods to make a nutritious morning shake.

Day 8: Meal Prep for the Work Week When trying to lose weight, it's especially important to plan and prepare your meals in advance, especially during the busy work week. You will be less likely to use the drive-thru on your way to work or to postmate an impulsive takeout order after a long day if you have healthy meals prepared and ready to enjoy. Set a goal for yourself to prepare options for breakfast, lunch, and snacks for the upcoming week! Can you keep doing this for the next thirty days? A little dedicated time for meal preparation is priceless.

Easy-to-Prepare Breakfast Options Make Blueberry Almond Overnight Oats or any other flavor you like. Make Egg Muffins with your favorite greens and vegetables. Make make-ahead smoothie packs and put them in the blender when you need a quick and easy healthy option. Easy-to-Prepare Lunch Options Make this meal-prep-friendly Veggie & Chickpea Pasta Salad and enjoy it hot or cold.

Make a protein-packed Peanut Butter Bliss Ball for an at-the-office snack or an on-the-go pre- or post-workout energy boost. Make a simple healthy hummus or guacamole and pack a serving to enjoy with sliced vegetables.

Day 9: Sleep for eight hours Did you know that getting enough sleep can help you lose weight? That is correct; getting less sleep has an impact on more than just your energy and mood! A minimum of eight hours of sleep could help you achieve your weight loss goals, according to research. How so? Putting more time on the pillow can help you burn more calories—those who sleep 8.5 hours or more on average burn 270 calories per night!

What about, on the other hand, lack of sleep? Not very good. It can set off hormonal imbalances, like more cortisol, a stress hormone that makes you gain weight. Leptin, your satiety hormone, will decrease and ghrelin, your hunger hormone, will rise when you don't get enough sleep.

Sleep deprivation can make it hard to lose weight. Try to prioritize this healthy habit tonight, throughout this challenge, and beyond!

Day 10: Aside from weight loss, it's important to move your body regularly. Plan your weekly workout schedule. Make time to plan your weekly workout schedule for today's challenge. Try to exercise three to five times per week, alternating between cardio, strength training, and recovery days. Make plans for your workouts just like you would for a meeting or appointment! The better it is, the more precise you can be.

You'll be more likely to stick to your workout schedule if you plan it out in advance. The advantages? You'll build lean muscle mass, speed up your metabolism, and burn more calories!

Day 11: Try calling on healthy food swaps rather than restricting your diet and eliminating your favorite foods! Today, focus solely on one food or ingredient. You might substitute fruit-infused water or a probiotic-rich seltzer for your usual soda. Instead of the sugar-laden store-bought creamer you typically enjoy, you might make your own. You might substitute a healthier version of your favorite pasta dish with chickpea pasta.

Start with just one or two food substitutions rather than attempting to completely alter your diet. Add one more when you feel stable! You'll have made dozens of manageable healthy substitutions before you know it. This is the key to making changes that last.

The following are some food substitutions that can help you lose weight:

Make your own nut or seed-based milk or creamer in place of dairy milk. Swap sugary soda for herbal iced tea, seltzer, cold-pressed juice, or coconut water. Mash avocado in place of mayo, butter, and cream cheese. Spiralize vegetables like zucchini, carrots, and squash in place of spaghetti and processed pasta. As you may be aware, mindfulness meditation is one of the best stress management strategies. While there are many reasons why chronic stress is bad, stress can make it hard to reach your weight loss goals.

The bright side? Emotions that may be preventing you from achieving your goals can be recognized and acknowledged without judgment, guilt, or shame through mindful meditation. Despite its apparent simplicity, do not underestimate its effectiveness! It has been demonstrated to be helpful for maintaining healthy eating and lifestyle habits as well as long-term weight loss.

Day 13: We are not suggesting that you have to give up alcohol completely (unless that is your goal). Instead, try a mock-tail instead. A healthy lifestyle can include the occasional drink, provided that it is enjoyed in moderation. However, abstaining from alcohol could be beneficial to your mind, body, and weight loss goals!

Alcohol is primarily devoid of additional nutrients and contains 7 calories per gram, making it a concentrated source of calories. And let's face it: once you start drinking, it's easy to overdo it.

But don't worry; you won't be left out! Cocktails can be replaced with mock-tails in a great way. Additionally, they are extremely delicious! There is a healthy mock-tail for every favorite drink, from Moscow mules to margaritas. The Watermelon Mint Cooler serves: 1 Components:

Crushed ice, 12 ounces unsweetened watermelon juice, 12 ounces sparkling or seltzer water, 1-2 tablespoons freshly squeezed lime juice, and fresh mint, according to taste Directions:

Step 1: Crushed ice should be added to the glass.

Step 2: Ice is topped with watermelon and lime juice.

Step 3: Add sparkling water to the top and stir to combine.

Step 4: Use fresh mint and lime to garnish. Enjoy!

Day 14: Avoid Added Sugars Now that you have completed two weeks, it is time to address a major issue: sugar! You are not alone if you struggle to cut back on sugar consumption because it is so addictive.

Read the ingredient label on everything to get started! Sugar can be found in more packaged foods than you might think, from pasta sauce to salad dressing. Start cutting out these foods and replacing them with healthier alternatives. It is not necessary to completely avoid sugar; however, if you must consume it, limit your consumption to whole-food sugar sources.

The least processed and healthiest options include fruit, raw honey, Medjool dates, and coconut sugar!

Day 15: Protein should come first—at every meal!

Protein is one of those nutrients that are good for you and is always a good idea, especially if you want to lose weight. It aids in the reduction of hunger pangs, boosts metabolism, and increases lean muscle mass—three crucial aspects of weight loss! Today, try to include protein in every meal.

Here are a few concepts:

A tablespoon of nut or seed butter can be added to your smoothie or oatmeal bowl. Top your salad with lean protein like grilled salmon, chicken, or tofu. Chia seeds can be added to overnight oats or baked goods. Greek yogurt can be added to sauces, dips, and spreads. Snack on hard-boiled eggs with vegetables or avocado.

Day 16: Eat until You're Full When your meal is packed full of delicious food, it can be tempting to lick your plate clean and savor each and every bite. Even if you're feeling full, you don't have to finish your plate! Remember: You can always save your food for later enjoyment because it won't disappear.

Instead, make an effort to chew your food, eat slowly, and stop when you are eighty percent full. You should be content, not full! Give this a shot today and see how it goes.

This trick for losing weight is a part of mindful eating, which has many benefits (more on this below). Try to pay attention to your own hunger cues and how you feel.

Day 17: Try a New Healthy Recipe It's easy to get bogged down in the same old cooking routine. Let's face it: it's easy and convenient to eat the same foods. However, if you're bored with your meals, you'll be more likely to reach for those tempting snacks. Additionally, if you stick with the same foods, you won't get all of the nutrients you need!

Today, try something completely different, whether it's something completely out of the ordinary or a recipe you've been meaning to try but haven't. Try doing this once a week. It will motivate you in the kitchen, provide you with a variety of nutrients, and introduce you to new foods. You can even make it a family affair by inviting your partner or kids to participate.

Day 18: Give Your Favorite Dessert a Healthy Makeover Sweet toothers, pay attention! Dessert can still help you lose weight. In point of fact, having a treat every now and then can assist in avoiding binges that are brought on by excessive dieting and food restriction. Having said that, if you want to satisfy your sweet tooth, you don't have to eat a lot of sugar, fat, or calories. There are numerous ways to transform your favorite treat into a guilt-free treat made with healthy ingredients.

Make a healthy cookie dough froyo with ingredients like Greek yogurt, almond butter, and cacao nibs. Roll up some no-bake bliss balls and enjoy one or two as a healthier alternative to cookies.

Day 19: Blend a naturally sweetened banana nice cream. Enjoy a 4-ingredient chocolate avocado pudding instead of the traditional high-sugar pudding. Make a Nutrient-Packed Smoothie Smoothies are a delicious and easy way to pack a lot of nutrients into a single meal or snack that only takes a few minutes to prepare. To make a meal that will help you lose weight, mix in some greens, a spoonful of super foods, and some hidden vegetables like cauliflower or zucchini.

Instead of eating one of the meals for today, try this Protein-Packed Banana Berry Fit On Smoothie!

Ingredients:

1 cup frozen berries, 1 cup oats, 1 tablespoon peanut butter, 3 cups Greek yogurt, 112 cups unsweetened almond milk, 1 chopped banana, and 2 teaspoons honey

Step 1: The oats should be added to the blender and pulsed a few times to make a fine flour. Blend in the remaining components until smooth. Taste and make any necessary changes to the ingredients.

Day 20: Join a Fitness Challenge

Now that you've been on this weight loss challenge for nearly three weeks, it's normal to lose steam. However, instead of giving up, try something new! Take on this 10-Day Kick starter Challenge if you're looking for some fresh exercise inspiration. In order to complete this challenge, you must complete ten workouts in ten days. You can even invite your friends to compete with you for fun. a great way to keep yourself accountable and motivated.

Are you ready to up your healthy eating game?

Whitney English's The Mindful Eater: a two-week program to help you get off diets. It simplifies nutrition!

Mona Sharma can reprogram your diet for you: a four-week program that will change how you lose weight for life.

Cara Clark's 101 Healthy Eating Tips: Say goodbye to food guilt, complicated regulations, and restrictions. Your mind and body will be transformed from the inside out during this four-week course!

Day 21: Develop an abundance mindset and think about the foods you can include instead of focusing on what to avoid. Eat the rainbow! A healthy and long-lasting method for losing weight is to include a lot of nutrients from whole foods that come in a variety of colors. Try to eat the rainbow for today's challenge. This means that you should eat as many different colored vegetables and fruits as you can; the more colors you have, the more nutrients you'll get!

Vegetables and fruits with red hues: high in quercetin and lycopene, which help maintain healthy skin, lower blood pressure, improve heart health, and support joints.

Orange and yellow fruits and vegetables: high in lutein and beta carotene, which support eye and skin health, improve immune health, and reduce the risk of chronic illness.

Vegetables and fruits that are blue or purple: high in flavonoids, anthocyanins, and resveratrol, which aid in healthy aging, heart health, and brain function.

Vegetables and fruits that are green: Sulforaphane, chlorophyll, and antioxidants help the body detoxify, boost digestion, and protect against free radical damage.

Vegetables and fruits that are white: abundant in anthoxanthins, antioxidants, and allicin.

Day 22: Pay Attention to Your Portion Sizes Although you are not required to begin tracking your macronutrients or calories, paying attention to your portion sizes is a great way to keep track of your serving sizes in a healthy and sustainable manner. It can help you avoid overeating, which is easy to do when you snack out of a bag or just spoon food onto your plate without thinking!

Try using your hand as a guide instead of fancy measuring cups or scales!

Day 23: One palm equals one serving of protein, one fist equals one serving of vegetables, one cupped hand equals one serving of carbs, and one thumb equals one serving of fat. Always carry a water bottle with you!

Water is your best friend when it comes to losing weight. Make sure you always have a reusable water bottle with you! It will act as a constant reminder to drink, which can help prevent overeating, quell sugar cravings, speed up metabolism, and make you feel fuller for longer.

Day 24: Avoid Eating While Distracted If you are accustomed to eating while working, walking, driving, or watching television, we challenge you to make a change! Overeating while distracted can occur immediately and later in the day! You'll feel less full and more likely to snack on unhealthy foods as a result. So, put your phone down, turn off your television, close your laptop, and sit down!

Mindful eating has been shown to reduce food cravings and reduce the amount of food consumed during meals, both of which are positive factors in weight loss.

Day 25: Become a Smart Snacker Are snacks preventing you from achieving your weight loss objectives? You won't be alone! However, the act of snacking is not always the issue. Instead, it depends on what kind of snacks you choose and how much you eat of them! We're thinking of processed chips, sugary cereals, pints of ice cream at midnight, and so on.

Take on the challenge of becoming a smart snacker. Choose whole-food snacks that are high in fiber, protein, and healthy fats rather than overindulging in foods high in calories but low in nutrients. And divide them up!

Some options:

Energy balls made with nut butter, oats, flax, and chia seeds Hard-boiled eggs with mashed avocado on the side Rice cakes with veggies, hummus, and a sprinkle of hemp seeds A protein-packed snack plate with nuts, edamame, and fruit or vegetables on the side Make Your Bedroom a Haven for Sleeping Remember what we said about getting enough sleep to lose weight? Well, sleep quality is just as important as sleep quantity when it comes to supporting your goals! Make your bedroom your haven for restful sleep.

Utilize a sound machine or earplugs to block out outside noise and maintain a cool temperature between 60 and 67 degrees Fahrenheit. Dim the lights, wear an eye mask, and turn off electronics.

Keep it clean because a messy place can make you anxious and make it hard to sleep!

Day 27: Change The Menu When Dining Out Don't be afraid to change the menu when dining out or placing an order! Healthy substitutions are readily accepted by restaurants, and they may even offer healthy alternatives that are not on the menu. Think: mashed avocado in place of calorie-rich dressings, gluten- or dairy-free pizza crusts and toppings, or non-dairy milk or creamer. Always pay attention to the ingredients and try to stick with whole-food alternatives!

Consider these healthy menu hacks to help you reach your weight loss goals:

Ask for sauces and dressings on the side, or substitute healthier alternatives like lemon juice, avocado, or a simple drizzle of olive oil. Choose oven-baked or grilled over fried. If possible, choose unsweetened. Ask if the food is gluten-free, dairy-free, or sugar-free. alternatives or whole-food alternatives When at all possible, stick to real, whole foods!

Day 28: When you're serving your food, make vegetables the star of your plate! They are low in calories, full of phytonutrients, low in sugar, and high in fiber. Choose non-starchy vegetables like zucchini, broccoli, kale, and spinach to fill half of your plate. You'll feel fuller for longer while getting a lot of nutrients into your body, which is a win-win situation!

Day 29: Warming Herbal Tea to End the Day Swap your late-night sweet snack for a cup of herbal tea! It has been demonstrated that some herbal teas improve digestion, speed up metabolism, and aid in weight loss. Therefore, go ahead and sip all day! However, if you're drinking it as a nightcap, check to see that it doesn't contain any caffeine before you pour it.

Some blends to think about: Dandelion leaf, ginger, oolong, rooibos, or matcha tea.

Day 30: Check in on your goals and write down how you feel about accomplishing them. 30 days of small, doable habits to help you reach your weight loss goals and stay there. Take a look back over the past month with a pen and paper.

5

CONSIDER JOURNALISM BY ASKING YOURSELF THE FOLLOWING QUESTIONS

What's going on?(Questions)

Consider your "why" and determine whether your driving force for weight loss has changed. Have your objectives evolved? How do they stack up to your goals from Day 1?

What really performed well? What modifications would you make?

How did you deal with your greatest source of stress during this challenge?

Which healthy routines have had the greatest effect on your day-to-day activities?

Make a list of your top five learnings. Are there any habits or areas you want to work on? Write them down. One of the most important keys to long-term weight loss is consistent self-reflection. Write down three to five positive affirmations and take the time to acknowledge your progress, no matter how small it may be. It aids in maintaining your intentionality, motivation, and focus. In addition, it

enables you to concentrate on your objectives and fine-tune any aspects that require enhancement or modification. It is more likely that you will complete your objectives, both long-term and short-term, if you return to your goals and your "why."

6

KEEP GOING

Continue on!

In the past thirty days, you've accomplished a lot; don't stop there! Make use of these easy ways to lose weight by incorporating them into your daily routine. You even have the option of repeating this challenge and starting from scratch! Take pride in your accomplishments. Remember: It's an adventure!

7

CONCLUSION

Dieting is one of those endeavors that almost invariably results in short-term failure. In point of fact, people who "diet" tend to gain more weight over time. Rather than concentrating solely on losing weight, make it your primary objective to provide your body with nutritious food.

Eat for health, happiness, and fitness, not just to lose weight.

Corpulence is a risky condition that is connected to various well-being results. Managing this condition is urgent to advancing great well-being and guaranteeing a decent personal satisfaction for everyone. Heftiness can be crushed by embraced a get-healthy plan. Getting thinner is an attractive and feasible objective that anyone can accomplish. In any case, a great many people expect that terrible weight is a difficult undertaking that is difficult to accomplish. This isn't the case,a individual can accomplish his/her objective of weight reduction. The excursion to weight reduction starts by having a feeling of assurance and demand.

From that point onward, the individual ought to hydrate, which will help in the decrease of how much food devoured. Smart dieting is significant to weight reduction, and this step ought to be finished to advance weight reduction and great well-being . At long last, the individual ought to participate in some actual activity. Through these means, the apparently intense test of getting in shape can be survived. The singular will actually want to accomplish a sound weight and stay away from every one of the unfortunate results related with stoutness.